PUBLIC HEALTH EMERGENCY RESPONSE GUIDE

FOR

STATE, LOCAL, AND TRIBAL PUBLIC HEALTH DIRECTORS

Version 2.0
April 2011

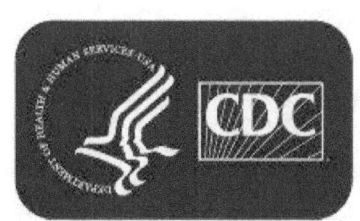

**U.S. Department of
Health and Human Services**
Centers for Disease
Control and Prevention

This guide is intended to assist state, local, and tribal public health professionals in the initiation of response activities during the first 24 hours of an emergency or disaster. It should be used in conjunction with existing emergency operations plans, procedures, guidelines, resources, assets, and incident management systems. It is not a substitute for public health emergency preparedness and planning activities. The response to any emergency or disaster must be a coordinated community effort.

CDC Emergency Response Hotline (24 Hours)

(770) 488-7100

This page intentionally left blank

TABLE OF CONTENTS

This page intentionally left blank

INTRODUCTION

This guide is intended to be used by state, local, and tribal public health professionals who are responsible for initiating public health response activities during the **first 24 hours** (i.e., the acute phase) of an emergency or disaster. It should be maintained by, and kept with, its primary user at all times. A small blank notebook or writing pad should be kept with this guide at all times to record thoughts and ideas generated through the use of the guide during the response to an incident. This guide is not intended to replace existing emergency operations plans, procedures, or guidelines. It is consistent with the doctrine, concepts, principles, terminology, organizational processes, and guidance in the *National Response Framework (NRF)* and the *National Incident Management System (NIMS).*

The guide begins with a brief section on public health emergency preparedness assumptions. The next section provides guidance and information on public health emergency response actions that should be initiated during the first 24 hours of an incident. This section is divided into three response timeframes: Immediate (hours 0-2), Intermediate (hours 2-6 and 6-12), and Extended (hours 12-24). The final section of the guide lists ongoing public health functions and tasks that should be considered beyond the first 24 hours of the response to an incident.

The guide concludes with five blank templates for your use:

Template 1 allows for the documentation of contacts and activities during the response to an incident.

Template 2 allows for the listing of contact information for key personnel within your health department. It should be completed by the user prior to an incident.

Template 3 allows for the listing of contact information for state, local, and tribal response partners within your community. It should be completed by the user prior to an incident.

Template 4 allows for the documentation of public health leadership assignments during the response to an incident.

Template 5 enables health departments to rank their level of preparedness to respond to specific types of incidents.

PUBLIC HEALTH EMERGENCY PREPAREDNESS ASSUMPTIONS

To effectively respond to an emergency or disaster, health departments must engage in preparedness activities. Completion of the following activities prior to an incident is essential to a successful response effort:

✓ Establish close working relationships and mutual-aid agreements with:
  - Emergency Management Agencies (EMAs)
  - Emergency Medical Services (EMS)
  - Medical/health/behavioral care providers
  - Fire, law enforcement, and other federal, state, local, and tribal response organizations
  - Local Emergency Planning Committees (LEPCs)
  - State, regional, and tribal public health response coordinators
  - Neighboring health jurisdictions
  - Humanitarian/non-governmental/ volunteer organizations
  - Community Emergency Response Teams (CERTs)
  - Medical Reserve Corps (MRC)
  - Private businesses
  - Academic institutions (schools of public health, medicine, nursing, etc.)
  - Other pertinent agencies/organizations

✓ Participate in hazard vulnerability and risk assessments for your area(s).

✓ Conduct a capacity assessment defining the resources of the public health system in your community and those available through mutual-aid agreements.

✓ Acquire resources and surge capacity necessary to perform the basic missions assigned to public health.

✓ Develop plans, procedures, and guidelines that are consistent with those used by other response agencies and organizations in your community.* Examples include:
  • All-hazards emergency operations plan
  • Incident-specific annexes**
  • Volunteer coordination guidelines
  • Health department staff assignments
  • Communication plans
  • Individual/family care plans
  • Command and management systems and authorities
  • Continuity of operations plan (COOP)

✓ Develop operational objectives for public health emergency response.

✓ Develop basic systems for morbidity, mortality, syndromic, and mental/behavioral surveillance, and registries for affected populations, with appropriate data archiving systems.

---

* *Should be consistent with the doctrine, concepts, principles, terminology, organizational processes, and guidance in the National Response Framework (NRF), National Incident Management System (NIMS), and FEMA Comprehensive Preparedness Guide (CPG) 101.*

** *For incident-specific preparedness, see* **Template 5,** *and the FEMA CPG 101*

✓ Develop plans, procedures, and guidelines for public affairs and risk communication.

✓ Engage in resource typing and credentialing of personnel, resources, and assets for emergency response.*

✓ Ensure that public health personnel within your department are trained and certified in safety and health practices, including the use of Personal Protective Equipment (PPE) for designated personnel. Consider on-scene credentialing.

✓ Provide orientation and training to public health response personnel, including volunteers, on the emergency operations plans, procedures, guidelines, command and management systems and authorities, and incident management system used by your community.

✓ Participate in the planning, design, and conduct of exercises to evaluate public health preparedness and response.***

✓ Participate in after-action reviews of exercises and actual incidents to identify areas that require revision, enhancement, and/or training, and take appropriate follow-up action through corrective action planning.***

***Should be consistent with the doctrine, concepts, principles, processes, and guidance in the Homeland Security Exercise and Evaluation Program (HSEEP)

This page intentionally left blank

PUBLIC HEALTH EMERGENCY RESPONSE FUNCTIONS AND TASKS DURING THE ACUTE PHASE

This section provides guidance and information on response activities that should be initiated during the first 24 hours (i.e., the acute phase) of most emergencies and disasters. Specific functions and tasks are divided into three response timeframes: **Immediate, Intermediate, and Extended.** The order in which these activities are undertaken may vary according to the specific incident, particularly during a biological incident or infectious disease outbreak. Because emergency response is a dynamic process, these activities may be repeated at various stages of the response.

Your health department should function as part of a larger overall emergency response effort. In most instances, your health department will not take the lead in responding to an incident. Your health department should always function within the emergency operations plans, procedures, guidelines, and incident management system used by your community.

The following guidance and information should be used as a reference until existing emergency operations plans, procedures, and guidelines are accessed. Each function and task outlined in the following sections of the guide should be accomplished in accordance with existing emergency operations plans, procedures, and guidelines.

11

Immediate Response: Hours 0 – 2

1. Assess the situation

Initiate the response by assessing the situation. Ask yourself the following questions and use a small blank notebook, writing pad, or other appropriate form(s) to record thoughts and ideas:

- Should public health become involved in the response? If so, in what way(s)?
- What public health function(s) has been or may be adversely impacted?
- What geographical area(s) has been or may be adversely impacted? Does it fall within your health department's jurisdiction?
- How many people are threatened, affected, exposed, injured, or dead?
- What are the exposure pathways?
- Have critical infrastructures been affected (e.g., electrical power, water supplies, sanitation, telecommunications, transportation, etc.)? If so, in what way(s)?
- Have medical and healthcare facilities been affected? If so, in what way(s)?
- Have public health operations been affected? If so, in what way(s)?
- Are escape routes open and accessible?
- How will current and forecasted weather conditions affect the situation?

- What other agencies and organizations are currently responding to the incident?
- What response actions have already been taken?
- Has information been communicated to responders and the public to protect public health? If so, in what way(s) and by whom?
- Does your health department have existing mutual-aid agreements with other agencies, organizations, or jurisdictions?
- Has an Incident Command Post (ICP) been established? If so, where is it?
- Who is the Incident Commander (IC)? How can the IC be contacted?
- Has the local, state, or tribal Emergency Operations Center (EOC) been activated? If so, where is it operating?

2. Contact key health personnel

Contact personnel within your health department that have emergency response roles and responsibilities. Examples include:

- Administration/Leadership
- Emergency Response Coordinators
- Environmental Health Specialists
- Epidemiologists
- Safety and Health Specialists
- Laboratory Personnel
- Mental and Behavioral Health Personnel
- Medical Officers/Nurses

- Public Information Officer (PIO)
- Medical Examiners/Coroners
- Animal Control Personnel
- Liaisons
- Technical, logistical, and other support personnel

Coordinate with other healthcare providers as necessary. Record all contacts, including unsuccessful attempts, and follow-up actions.

3. Develop initial health response objectives and establish an action plan

Develop initial health response objectives that are specific, measurable, achievable, and time-framed. Establish an action plan based on your assessment of the situation. Assign responsibilities and record all actions.

4. Public health participation in the Emergency Operations Center (EOC)

A health representative(s) from your department should be assigned to establish communications and maintain close coordination with the local, state, or tribal EOC and its associated components, if operational. The health representative(s) may or may not be physically located in the EOC depending on the specific incident and established emergency operations plans, procedures, and guidelines.

14

5. Ensure that the site health and safety plan (HASP) is established, reviewed, and followed

Coordinate with the safety officer to identify hazards or unsafe conditions associated with the incident and immediately alert and inform appropriate supervisors and leadership personnel. This can be achieved through site safety briefings and at shift changes. Responder safety and health reports, updates, and briefings should be initiated at this stage of the response. Ensure that medical personnel are available to evaluate and treat response personnel.

6. Establish communications with key health and medical organizations

Establish communications with other health and medical agencies, facilities, and organizations that have emergency response roles and responsibilities, and verify their treatment and support capacities (e.g., patient isolation and/or decontamination, etc.) Examples include:

- Emergency Medical Services (EMS)
- Hospitals and clinics
- Laboratories
- Nursing homes/assisted living facilities
- Home health care agencies
- Psychiatric/mental/behavioral health and social services providers

- State and county medical societies
- Liaisons (to special populations, etc.)
- Other health and medical entities, as appropriate

Record all contacts, including unsuccessful attempts, and any follow-up actions.

REMINDER!

See **Template 1** at the back of the guide to document the contacts you make and any follow-up actions during the incident. See **Templates 2 and 3** at the back of the guide for emergency contact information specific to your health department and jurisdiction.

---

7. Assign and deploy resources and assets to achieve established initial health response objectives

Many objectives may not be achieved immediately during the response. Effective allocation and monitoring of health resources and assets will be required to sustain 24-hour response operations.

REMINDER!

Use **Template 4** at the back of the guide to document public health leadership assignments during the response to an incident.

---

8. Address requests for assistance and information

As part of the community response effort, ensure that health-related requests for assistance and information from other agencies, organizations, and the public are either directed to appropriate personnel within your health department or forwarded to appropriate agencies and organizations.

9. Initiate risk communication activities

Determine whether a Joint Information Center (JIC) and the local, state, or tribal Emergency Operations Center (EOC) are operational. If so, ensure that a health representative(s) from your department has been assigned as part of a Joint Information System (JIS) to establish communications and maintain close coordination with the JIC. The health representative(s) may or may not be physically located in the JIC based on the specific incident and established emergency operations plans, procedures, and guidelines.

Ensure that contact has been established with appropriate personnel within your health department and initiate risk communication activities. Remember to communicate public health messages in the appropriate language(s) to persons with limited English proficiency. A public health information "hotline" can be established to address requests for information from the public.

REMINDER!

Preparing Messages

Employ the STARCC Principle

Your public message in a crisis must be:

Simple . . .   Frightened people don't want to hear big words

Timely . . .   Frightened people want information NOW

Accurate . . .   Frightened people won't get nuances so give it straight

Relevant . . .   Answer their questions and give action steps

Credible . . .   Empathy and openness are key to credibility

Consistent . . .   The slightest change in the message is upsetting and dissected by all

Source: Reynolds, B., Crisis and Emergency Risk Communication by Leaders for Leaders. Atlanta, GA: Centers for Disease Control and Prevention, 2004

REMINDER!

Delivering Messages

When engaging in risk communication, build trust and credibility by expressing . . .

- Empathy and caring
- Competence and expertise
- Honesty and openness
- Commitment and dedication

Top tips . . .

- Don't over reassure
- Acknowledge uncertainty
- Express wishes ("I wish I had answers")
- Explain the process in place to find answers
- Acknowledge people's fear
- Give people things to do
- Ask more of people (share risk)

As a spokesperson . . .

- Know your organization's policies
- Stay within the scope of responsibilities
- Tell the truth. Be transparent
- Embody your agency's identity

CONSISTENT MESSAGES ARE VITAL!

Source: Reynolds, B., Crisis and Emergency Risk Communication. Atlanta, GA: Centers for Disease Control and Prevention, 2002.

10. Engage legal counsel as part of the emergency response effort

Stay apprised of legal issues as they emerge and consult with appropriate personnel within your health department and jurisdiction.

11. Document all response activities

Document all response activities using the form(s) within your health department. **Templates 1 and 4** at the back of the guide can also assist with the documentation of initial response activities.

This page intentionally left blank

Intermediate Response: Hours 2 – 6

REMINDER!

As part of the community response effort, continue to perform the following activities:

✓   Assess the situation

✓   Review and update health response objectives

✓   Review, update, and follow the site health and safety plan (HASP)

✓   Communicate with key health and medical agencies/organizations and neighboring jurisdictions

✓   Address requests for assistance and information

✓   Continue risk communication activities

✓   Stay apprised of legal issues

✓   Document all response activities

INITIATE THE FOLLOWING ACTIVITIES:

1. Verify that health surveillance systems are operational

Health surveillance systems should be fully operational to begin the process of data collection and analysis. Consider human subjects and privacy issues related to data collection, analysis, and storage.

2. Ensure that laboratories likely to be used during the response are operational and verify their analytical capacity

Laboratories likely to be used during the response should be fully operational to begin the process of specimen collection and analysis. Notify laboratories of any changes in activity during the response. Provide laboratories with lead time to prepare for sample testing and analysis.

3. Ensure that the needs of special populations are being addressed

Ensure that the needs of special populations are being addressed through the provision of appropriate information and assistance. Examples of special populations include:

- Children
- Dialysis patients

- Disabled persons
- Homebound patients
- Patients dependent on home health care services
- Institutionalized persons
- Persons with limited English proficiency
- The elderly
- Transient populations (tourists, migrant workers, the homeless, carnival/fair workers, etc.)

4. Health-related volunteers and donations

Communicate frequently with the public regarding whether or not health-related volunteers and donations are needed. Volunteer agencies (e.g., the Red Cross) have their own needs that may differ from those of your health department. Volunteer medical personnel must be properly credentialed and insured.

5. Update risk communication messages

Ensure that risk communication messages are updated and coordinated with other responding agencies and organizations as necessary. If a Joint Information Center (JIC) is operational, update and release messages through the JIC. Ensure that messages on public health information "hotlines" are updated as necessary.

This page intentionally left blank

Intermediate Response: Hours 6 – 12

REMINDER!

As part of the community response effort, continue to perform the following activities:

✓   Assess the situation

✓   Review and update health response objectives

✓   Communicate with key health and medical agencies organizations and neighboring jurisdictions

✓   Address requests for assistance and information

✓   Continue risk communication activities

✓   Stay apprised of legal issues

✓   Communicate with health surveillance and laboratory contacts

✓   Address the needs of special populations

✓   Organize health-related volunteers and donations

✓   Document all response activities

INITIATE THE FOLLOWING ACTIVITIES:

1. Collect and analyze data that are becoming available through health surveillance and laboratory systems

Begin collecting and analyzing data that are becoming available through established health surveillance systems and laboratories, and evaluate any real-time sampling data. Communicate results to appropriate personnel in a timely manner through established operations plans, procedures, or guidelines.

2. Prepare and update information for shift change and executive briefings

Initiate staffing plan and update contact information and rosters to be used by incoming personnel. Apprise incoming personnel of response actions being taken, pending decisions and issues, deployment of resources and assets, updated health response objectives, and current media activities.

3. Prepare for state and federal on-site assistance

Prepare for the arrival of state and federal on-site assistance and for the integration of these personnel, resources, and assets into the locally established response structure. Examples include:

- Technical experts and Emergency Response Coordinators (ERCs)
- U.S. Department of Health and Human Services (HHS) Incident Response Coordination Team (IRCT)
- Centers for Disease Control and Prevention (CDC) personnel
- Strategic National Stockpile (SNS)
- Federal Medical Station (FMS)
- Environmental Response Team (ERT)
- U.S. Environmental Protection Agency (EPA) Radiological Emergency Response Team (RERT)
- Veterans Health Administration (VHA) Medical Emergency Radiology Response Team (MERRT)
- Federal Radiological Monitoring and Assessment Center (FRMAC) personnel
- National Disaster Medical System (NDMS) Teams:
  — Disaster Medical Assistance Team (DMAT)
  — National Medical Response Team (NMRT)
  — Disaster Mortuary Operational Response Team (DMORT)
  — National Veterinary Response Team (NVRT)

- U.S. Public Health Service (USPHS) Commissioned Corps Teams
  — Rapid Deployment Force (RDF)
  — Applied Public Health Team (APHT)
  — Mental Health Team (MHT)
- Administration for Children and Families (ACF) Disaster Case Managment (DCM) Teams
- Personnel, equipment, resources, and assets via the Emergency Management Assistance Compact (EMAC)
- Other specialized response teams

4. Assess health resource needs and acquire as necessary

Resources and capacity to meet health response objectives must be reviewed periodically and appropriate action taken to ensure their availability. Effective allocation and monitoring of health resources and assets will be required to sustain 24-hour and extended response operations.

Extended Response: Hours 12 – 24

REMINDER!

As part of the community response effort, continue to perform the following activities:

✓ Assess the situation

✓ Review and update health response objectives

✓ Communicate with key health and medical agencies/organizations and neighboring jurisdictions

✓ Address requests for assistance and information

✓ Continue risk communication activities

✓ Stay apprised of legal issues

✓ Collect and analyze data through surveillance and laboratory systems

✓ Address the needs of special populations

✓ Organize health-related volunteers and donations

✓ Collaborate with state and federal on-site assistance

✓ Assess health resource needs and acquire as necessary

✓ Document all response activities

INITIATE THE FOLLOWING ACTIVITIES:

1. Address mental and behavioral health support needs

Initiate preparations for providing mental and behavioral health services, and social services, to health department staff, response personnel, and other persons affected by the event. Address required comfort needs of health department staff.

2. Prepare for transition to extended operations or response disengagement

Consider and assess public health functions and tasks that will need to be addressed beyond the first 24 hours (i.e., the acute phase) of the incident based on incoming data and developments. Your health department may be engaged in extended operations for lengthy periods of time. Also, begin developing a strategy for disengaging and demobilizing public health from the response effort based on the analysis and results of incoming data and existing response objectives.

ONGOING PUBLIC HEALTH EMERGENCY RESPONSE FUNCTIONS AND TASKS

This section provides a list of public health emergency response functions, tasks, and prevention services that may need to be implemented during an emergency or disaster beyond the first 24 hours (i.e., the acute phase) of the response. These activities should be considered regardless of the type of incident (i.e., natural or technological/man-made). The order in which these activities are undertaken may vary according to the specific incident, particularly during a biological incident or infectious disease outbreak, and geographic location. This information should be used as a reference until existing emergency operations plans, procedures, and guidelines are accessed.

✓ Environmental hazard identification

✓ Hazards consultation

✓ Epidemiological services

✓ Health and medical needs assessment

✓ Identification of affected individuals

✓ Contamination control

✓ Health surveillance

✓ Laboratory specimen collection and
    analysis

✓ Infectious disease identification, treatment,
    and control

✓ Quarantine/isolation

✓ Public health information

✓ Risk communication

✓ Responder safety and health

✓ Health and medical personnel resources

✓ Health and medical equipment safety and
    availability

✓ Health-related volunteer and donation
    coordination

✓ In-hospital care

✓ Evacuation

✓ Sheltering

✓ Special populations needs and assistance

✓ Mass trauma

✓ Mass fatalities

✓ Mortuary services

✓ Mental/behavioral health care and social services

✓ Potable water

✓ Food safety

✓ Vector control and pest management

✓ Wastewater and solid-waste management/disposal

✓ Building/facility assessment

✓ Sanitation/hygiene services

✓ Continuity of public health programs, services, and infrastructure

✓ Veterinary services

✓ Animal rescue/control/shelters

✓ Long-term community recovery

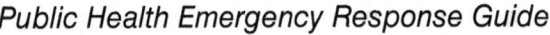

This page intentionally left blank

TEMPLATE 1. DOCUMENTATION OF CONTACTS AND ACTIONS

This template allows for the creation of a running log through the documentation of contacts made and response actions initiated during the initial hours of an incident until existing forms or logs are accessed. All contacts, including unsuccessful attempts, and follow-up actions should be recorded below. The initial resulting record can be used to identify particular areas in your emergency operations plan, procedures, or guidelines that may need revision.

Contacts	Date	Time	Actions/Comments

Contacts	Date	Time	Actions/Comments

Contacts	Date	Time	Actions/Comments

Contacts	Date	Time	Actions/Comments

TEMPLATE 2. HEALTH DEPARTMENT PERSONNEL EMERGENCY CONTACT INFORMATION

Record emergency contact information for key health department personnel in this section prior to an incident. Contact information can be inserted and updated by either using the following template or placing a self-adhesive label (e.g., Avery* 3259) or securing (e.g., taping) a 3"x5" note card or piece of paper with written/typed information in its place.

Name	Office/ Functional Area	Office #	Mobile/Pager #	E-mail

*Use of this trade name does not imply endorsement by the Centers for Disease Control and Prevention (CDC).

41

Name	Office/Functional Area	Office #	Mobile/Pager #	E-mail

TEMPLATE 3. STATE, LOCAL, AND TRIBAL EMERGENCY CONTACT INFORMATION

Record location-specific emergency contact information in this section prior to an incident. Contact information can be inserted and updated by either using the following template or placing a self-adhesive label (e.g., Avery* 3259) or securing (e.g., taping) a 3"x5" note card or piece of paper with written/typed information in its place.

Name	Office/ Functional Area	Office #	Mobile/Pager #	E-mail

Use of this trade name does not imply endorsement by the Centers for Disease Control and Prevention (CDC).

Name	Office/ Functional Area	Office #	Mobile/Pager #	E-mail

TEMPLATE 4. LEADERSHIP ASSIGNMENTS

This template allows for the documentation of health department leadership assignments made during the public health response to an incident. Not all assignments will necessarily be staffed due to variations in health department resources and response requirements for a particular incident. Blank space is provided at the end of the template to allow users to list additional locations and assignments as necessary.

Response Assignments		Assigned Leadership	Date & Time In/Out
Incident Command Post (ICP):	1.		
	2.		
Site Control	1.		
	2.		
Site Health/Safety	1.		
	2.		

Response Assignments		Assigned Leadership	Date & Time In/Out
Health Department Operations:	1.		
	2.		
Operations/ Command Center	1.		
	2.		
Field Operations	1.		
	2.		
Epidemiology Services	1.		
	2.		
Laboratory Support	1.		
	2.		
Information Systems	1.		
	2.		

Response Assignments		Assigned Leadership	Date & Time In/Out
Community Services	1.		
	2.		
Administrative Services	1		
	2		
Environmental Services	1		
	2.		
Communications	1.		
	2.		
Liaison(s)	1		
	2		

Response Assignments		Assigned Leadership	Date & Time In/Out
Emergency Operations Center (EOC):	1		
	2.		
Command	1		
	2		
Safety	1		
	2		
Liaison(s)	1		
	2.		
Planning	1		
	2		
Operations	1		
	2.		
Logistics	1		
	2		

Response Assignments		Assigned Leadership	Date & Time In/Out
Finance/ Administration	1		
	2		
Intelligence/ Investigations	1.		
	2.		
Joint Information System (JIS)	1.		
	2		
Joint Information Center (JIC)	1		
	2		
Joint Operations Center (JOC)	1.		
	2.		
Joint Field Office (JFO)	1.		
	2.		

Response Assignments	Assigned Leadership	Date & Time In/Out
Decontamination Site(s)	1.	
	2.	
Hospitals, clinics, and other medical facilities	1.	
	2.	
Strategic National Stockpile (SNS) receipt site(s)	1.	
	2.	
Vaccine/medicine distribution site(s)	1.	
	2.	
Shelter(s)	1.	
	2.	

Response Assignments	Assigned Leadership		Date & Time In/Out
	1.		
	2.		
	1.		
	2.		
	1.		
	2.		
	1.		
	2.		
	1.		
	2.		

This page intentionally left blank

TEMPLATE 5. INCIDENT-SPECIFIC PUBLIC HEALTH PREPAREDNESS

The following template can be used to help determine your health department's level of preparedness to respond to direct and indirect public health threats associated with specific types of emergencies and disasters. Incidents are divided into two categories: Natural and Technological/Man-made*. The incidents listed in this template are only examples and should not be considered all-inclusive. Blank space is provided at the end of the template to allow users to list additional incidents that may affect their area(s). Use the grid to evaluate your health department's ability to respond to specific incidents by placing an "X" next to each incident under the ranking that most accurately represents your health department's level of preparedness to respond to that particular incident. This evaluation should be based on state and local public health emergency preparedness guidance developed by CDC and the doctrine, concepts, principles, terminology, and organizational processes in the *National Response Framework (NRF)* and *National Incident Management System (NIMS)*. When completed, this template can be used to prioritize preparedness activities and can identify those incidents for which additional (state, federal, etc.) response assistance would be required. This template should be updated as new preparedness activities are undertaken.

* *Technological/Man-made incidents can be intentional or unintentional, including acts of terrorism.*

Ranking

Type of Incident	Most Prepared			Least Prepared		
	4	3	2	1	N/A
Natural					
Avalanche					
Drought					
Earthquake					
Extreme cold					
Extreme heat					

Ranking

Type of Incident	Most Prepared		Least Prepared		
	4	3	2	1	N/A
Natural					
Fire/Wildfire					
Flood					
Hurricane/ tropical storm					
Infectious disease outbreak					
Landslide/mudflow					

Ranking

Type of Incident	Most Prepared		Least Prepared		
	4	3	2	1	N/A
Natural					
Pandemic Influenza					
Snow/blizzard					
Thunderstorm/ lightning					
Tornado					
Tsunami					
Volcano					

Ranking

Type of Incident	Most Prepared 4	3	2	Least Prepared 1	N/A
Technological/Man-made					
Airplane crash					
Biological release					
Building/structural collapse					
Chemical/hazardous substance release					
Civil unrest/ disobedience					

Ranking

Type of Incident	Most Prepared 4	3	Least Prepared 2	1	N/A
Technological/Man-made					
Critical infrastructure failure:					
Telecommunications					
Electrical power					
Gas and oil					
Transportation					
Water supply					
Sanitation					

Ranking

Type of Incident	Most Prepared		Least Prepared		
	4	3	2	1	N/A
Technological/Man-made					
Explosion (conventional)					
Maritime					
Mass immigration					
Mass public gathering					
Mine collapse/explosion					

Ranking

Type of Incident	Most Prepared		Least Prepared		
	4	3	2	1	N/A
Technological/Man-made					
Radiological/nuclear					
Train derailment					

Ranking

Type of Incident	Most Prepared		Least Prepared		N/A
	4	3	2	1	
Other Incident					

This page intentionally left blank

Questions regarding this guide should be addressed to Martin A. Kalis with CDC's Environmental Health Services Branch (EHSB) at (770) 488-4568 or pherg@cdc.gov.

An electronic version of this guide can be downloaded from the CDC Emergency Preparedness and Response Web site at http://emergency.cdc.gov/planning/responseguide.asp.

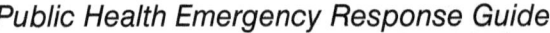

This page intentionally left blank